Study Guide to Accompany

Seventh Edition

OUR GLOBAL ENVIRONMENT

A Health Perspective

Anne Nadakavukaren

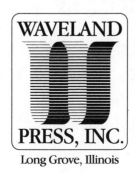
WAVELAND
PRESS, INC.
Long Grove, Illinois

For information about this book, contact:
  Waveland Press, Inc.
  4180 IL Route 83, Suite 101
  Long Grove, IL 60047-9580
  (847) 634-0081
  info@waveland.com
  www.waveland.com

10-digit ISBN 1-57766-727-1
13-digit ISBN 978-1-57766-727-8

Printed in the United States of America

8   7   6   5   4

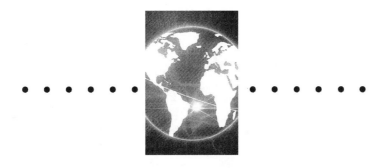

NOTE TO STUDENTS

The following pages of exercises, related to topics covered in the corresponding chapters of *Our Global Environment: A Health Perspective, Seventh Edition,* are intended as a means for reviewing text material and stimulating consideration of issues raised in your reading.

For maximum personal benefit, it is recommended that you first read the appropriate chapter, then attempt to answer as many questions as possible without reference to the book, and subsequently return to the text to complete any remaining items of which you are unsure.

• • • • • • • • 1 • • • • • • • •

Introduction to Ecological Principles

A. Match the following definitions with the correct terms:

_____ 1. environmental conditions that control where an organism can live

_____ 2. a relatively stable, self-perpetuating biotic community

_____ 3. a natural area where living things interact with the chemical and physical environment

_____ 4. animal species that moderate competition among prey species, thereby maintaining greater diversity within the community

_____ 5. the relative position occupied by an organism in a food chain

_____ 6. complex of communities characteristic of a regional climatic zone

_____ 7. gradual replacement of one biotic community by another over time

_____ 8. natural grouping of various plant and animal species within a given habitat

_____ 9. nonnative organisms introduced into an established biotic community

_____ 10. organisms that largely control the flow of energy through a community

_____ 11. individuals of the same species living together within a given area

_____ 12. adaptations to life in a specific environment that reduce competition among species for food and living space

a. ecological dominant

b. niche diversification

c. exotic species

d. succession

e. limiting factors

f. eutrophication

g. biotic community

h. ecosystem

i. trophic level

j. biome

k. climax community

l. population

m. keystone predator

n. biomass

B. True/False. If statement is false, revise it below in space provided to make a correct statement; focus your response on the words in bold.

_____ 1. A greater number of different plant and animal species can be found **in the taiga** than in a tropical rain forest.

_____ 2. In most biotic communities, certain **plants** comprise the ecological dominants.

_____ 3. Keystone predators **reduce biotic diversity by consuming large numbers of prey species.**

_____ 4. It would be accurate to refer to the **tundra** as a "cold desert."

_____ 5. "Boom-and-bust" cycles are a characteristic feature of the **temperate deciduous forest.**

_____ 6. **Desert and tundra** are two of the most fragile biomes—those where human pressures are likely to have very detrimental and long-lasting effects.

_____ 7. **Tropical rain forests** offer great promise as future world "breadbaskets" if their deep, rich topsoil could be exploited for agriculture.

_____ 8. An organism that has **a broad tolerance range for various limiting factors** will enjoy a wider geographic distribution than one with a narrow range of tolerance.

_____ 9. Consumer organisms are generally **more numerous and smaller in size** than are producer organisms.

_____ 10. The typical food chain consists of **no more than 4 or 5** trophic levels.

_____ 11. As energy is transferred within a food chain, **more** usable energy is available to the top predators than to primary consumers.

_____ 12. Trace elements are mineral nutrients that improve the vigor of plants but which, unlike the macronutrients, **are not absolutely essential for plant growth.**

_____ 13. Biogeochemical cycling helps to maintain the stability of ecosystems **by retaining vital nutrients in forms usable by plants and animals.**

_____ 14. Elements moving in **gaseous cycles** recycle more quickly and efficiently than do those characteristic of sedimentary cycles.

_____ 15. Unlike petroleum and coal, **phosphate deposits are renewable resources** whose supplies are constantly being replenished as organic tissues decompose and return to the soil.

_____ 16. Burmese pythons are thriving and multiplying in southern Florida largely thanks to **a climate change-induced rise in average temperature.**

_____ 17. The kelp "forest" ecosystem off the coast of Alaska is in danger of collapsing because **spills from oil tankers have poisoned the marine food chain.**

_____ 18. Through the process of ecological succession, lakes and ponds will eventually be transformed into **terrestrial climax communities**.

_____ 19. Accelerating the natural process of eutrophication would be **beneficial to human interests**.

_____ 20. The most ambitious environmental restoration effort ever attempted is now underway in **the Florida Everglades.**

C. List some representative plant and animal species in each of the following biomes and cite a major physical characteristic of each of those environments:

a. tropical rain forest

b. taiga

c. tundra

d. temperate deciduous forest

e. desert

f. grassland

7

D. Fill-in-the-Blank:

_____   1. Which biome is characterized by permanently frozen subsoil?

_____   2. In which biome is laterization of exposed soils a major obstacle to agricultural development?

_____   3. What is the evolutionary value in the tendency of populations to become increasingly specialized for life in a particular "ecological niche"?

_____   4. What is the ultimate energy source for all life activities?

a) _____   5. Cite two factors contributing to the forest devastation caused by mountain pine beetles in the western U.S. and Canada.

b) _____

_____   6. What is the primary cause of eutrophication?

_____   7. Name a food item whose consumption would make us tertiary consumers.

_____   8. What is the principal inorganic source of carbon available to living things?

_____   9. How is this form of carbon made available?

_____   10. Name one means by which atmospheric nitrogen can be incorporated into living tissues.

_____   11. Name an exotic species deliberately introduced in the southeastern U.S. for erosion control that is now a serious invasive weed.

_____   12. Give an example of a "pioneer plant."

_____   13. Cite a characteristic feature of pioneer plants that explains why they are the first organisms to colonize a previously barren area.

_____   14. Give an example of a place where you might observe secondary succession in progress.

a) _____   15. Cite one positive and one negative environmental impact of ecotourism.

b) _____

E. Essay:

Discuss some modern-day examples of human modification of an ecosystem with which you are familiar and cite some of the direct or indirect consequences such disruption has had on biotic communities and/or human populations.

F. Activity:

Measure off a piece of ground (quadrant) one yard square in an outdoor area of your choice.

a) Describe the abiotic components of that ecosystem and list the living organisms inhabiting the designated area.

b) Describe the interactions among members of that biotic community and the relationship between the physical environment and the life forms that you observe there.

c) Diagram one type of food chain operative within your quadrant, using specific organisms as examples of the different trophic levels.

• • • • • • • 2 • • • • • • • •

Population Dynamics

A. Fill-in-the-Blank:

_____ 1. Which region of the world is experiencing the highest rates of population growth?

_____ 2. In which region of the world has population growth essentially stabilized?

_____ 3. What is the present population of the world?

_____ 4. What is the current world growth rate?

_____ 5. At the current rate of growth, how long will it take for world population to double?

_____ 6. What is the population of the United States?

_____ 7. What is the population growth rate of the United States?

_____ 8. What variable, other than birth and death rates, will be an important determinant of the ultimate population size of the U.S.?

_____ 9. Name a country with a negative growth rate.

_____ 10. What country is currently the world's most populous nation?

_____ 11. What type of population profile is characteristic of a country with a rapidly growing population?

a) _____ 12. Name an industrialized country where the male death rate has sharply increased in recent decades. Cite one possible reason for this unfortunate trend.

b) _____

_____ 13. If a particular society had a birth rate of 38 and a death rate of 15, what would its growth rate be?

_____ 14. How many people live in a "megacity"?

_____ 15. Approximately what percentage of the world's people now live in urban areas?

_____ 16. What is considered a "high" birth rate?

15

B. Identify and explain the significance of each of the following:

1. Thomas Malthus

2. demographic transition

3. biotic potential

4. environmental resistance

5. carrying capacity

6. homeostatic control

7. doubling time

8. "global graying"

C. Short-Answer Questions:

1. Describe the S-curve and J-curve patterns of growth; what accounts for the difference between the two?

2. Give an example of an environment whose carrying capacity may already have been exceeded. Explain what is happening there.

3. What characteristic of the age structure in most developing countries will prevent a rapid stabilization of population size even in societies with vigorous family-planning programs?

4. What future problems/challenges confront societies in countries where population levels have stabilized or are decreasing? Give some specific examples.

5. Will the AIDS epidemic reverse the rapid increase in Africa's population growth? Explain the demographic impact of the disease.

6. Explain in demographic terms why the current "population explosion" is exclusively a developing world phenomenon.

7. How do high population growth rates contribute to "Failed States"?

Name _____

D. Activity:
Assume that the population of the United States continues to grow at its present rate throughout your life-time and that of your children and grandchildren. Under column A below list as many benefits of such growth as you can think of; under column B, list all the disadvantages additional growth might pose. What conclusions regarding the desirability of future growth do you draw from a comparison of your two lists?

A	B

Conclusions:

• • • • • • • 3 • • • • • • •

Population Control

A. Match the following birth control facts with the appropriate device or method (Note: the same answer may be used more than once):

_____ 1. most widely practiced method of birth control in the U.S. among women 15–44 who practice contraception

_____ 2. doctor's prescription needed to obtain this type of vaginal contraceptive

_____ 3. pelvic inflammatory disease is the most worrisome side effect of this contraceptive

_____ 4. a decline in the risk of ovarian and endometrial cancer is associated with use of this contraceptive

_____ 5. protection against sexually transmitted diseases is an additional benefit provided by this contraceptive

_____ 6. the safest and most reliable of all contraceptive methods

_____ 7. contraceptive administered as an injection every 3 months

_____ 8. contraceptive that is not recommended for women who have never been pregnant

_____ 9. ancient birth control technique still widely practiced; safe, but with high failure rate

_____ 10. women over 40 are advised not to use this method

_____ 11. a form of emergency contraception

_____ 12. malnourished or anemic women may experience difficulties with this contraceptive

_____ 13. women who smoke are cautioned not to use this method

_____ 14. a high level of motivation and cooperation between partners is required for this method's success

_____ 15. both safe and effective when used in combination with vaginal contraceptives

a. pill

b. IUD

c. sterilization

d. condom

e. withdrawal

f. natural family planning

g. sponge

h. foam/gels

i. diaphragm

j. Plan B

k. Depo-Provera

B. Fill-in-the-Blank:

a) _____

1. Give two reasons why withdrawal is still widely practiced in some cultures as a family limitation method.

b) _____

_____

2. How effective is breast-feeding in terms of protecting a woman against pregnancy?

_____

3. For what purpose were condoms originally intended?

_____

4. What is the main deterrent to sterilization as a method of birth control?

_____

5. Who is credited with launching the birth control movement in the U.S.?

_____

6. What has always been the primary goal of the American family-planning movement?

_____

7. Among sexually-active U.S. women at risk of an unwanted pregnancy, what percentage practice some form of birth control?

_____

8. Biologically, what is the optimum age range for child bearing?

_____

9. In what age group are women most likely to die due to complications of pregnancy or childbirth?

_____

10. The incidence of birth defects is highest among babies of women in which age category?

_____

11. After what age does a woman's ability to conceive begin to decline?

_____

12. Statistically, the risk of maternal death, miscarriage, stillbirth, or neonatal death begins to increase with which pregnancy?

_____

13. For what purpose are ultrasound scanners and amniocentesis being misused in some Asian countries?

_____

14. How does mifepristone differ from Plan B?

_____

15. How does the contraceptive effectiveness of the Ortho-Evra® patch compare with that of the pill?

_____

16. Postponing marriage and pregnancy for young girls would be the most effective way of preventing what tragic health problem related to childbirth in developing counties?

_____

17. What is the most popular method of birth control in the United States today?

_____   18. What population policy has the People's Republic of China adopted in an effort to stabilize its population size?

_____   19. What single factor did delegates to the 1994 U.N. Conference on Population and Development feel was most important in efforts to lower developing world fertility?

_____   20. Compare the safety and effectiveness of male vs. female sterilization.

C. Discussion Questions:

1. In terms of a good reproductive health program, why is a wide range of contraceptive options desirable? Give specific examples to illustrate your answer.

2. In what ways does the implementation of family-planning programs in developing countries differ from that in North America and Europe? Why is this difference in approach necessary for the success of such efforts?

3. Explain why it is difficult to convince many couples in the developing world to have fewer children. What do you feel would be the most effective approach to reducing their birth rates? Why?

4. Explain how Plan B can provide protection against unwanted pregnancy.

5. What factors account for the growing gap between male and female births in China and India? Why have government attempts to correct the situation been largely unsuccessful?

D. Exercise:

Interview 5–10 of your friends or acquaintances (preferably individuals who have not taken this class) to determine their extent of awareness and personal opinions on the following population-related questions:

Population Awareness Survey

1. What is your estimate of current world population size? U.S. population size?

2. Are you at all worried about world overpopulation? Why or why not?

3. Do you think the U.S. has a population problem? Explain.

4. Do you think overpopulation has any effect on you personally? If so, in what way?

5. What actions, if any, do you think the U.S. government should take to deal with this problem, either domestically or internationally?

6. What do you think is the best population size for the United States? (i.e., lower than at present? the same? higher?)

7. Do you feel any sense of personal responsibility for influencing world population problems through your own reproductive behavior? Explain your response.

8. How many children do you want to have? Why do you feel this is the appropriate number for you?

Discuss your reactions to the answers you received. Do you feel the respondents were well informed on the basic issues involved? Do you think the opinions expressed would have been substantially different if you had interviewed individuals of various ages or socioeconomic backgrounds? Did the replies you received make you more or less optimistic about humanity's prospects of stabilizing population size?

• • • • • • • • 4 • • • • • • • •

The People-Food Predicament

A. Short-Answer Questions:

1. List three factors largely responsible for the significant increase in North American food production since the end of World War II.

   a)

   b)

   c)

2. Describe the trends in world food production vis-a-vis population growth from 1950 to the present.

3. To what extent does expanding the amount of land under cultivation offer hope for significantly increasing world food supply? Why?

4. List four reasons for the loss of currently productive agricultural land.

   a)

   b)

   c)

   d)

39

5. What factors make it unlikely that ocean fish harvests can be increased substantially above present levels?

6. List several changes in food-handling practices that poor countries could implement to prevent loss of harvested crops.

7. To what extent can "eating lower on the food chain" help to solve problems of world hunger?

8. Why are a number of relatively affluent countries purchasing farmland in other nations? What are the advantages and disadvantages of such purchases for the host country?

B. Match the following deficiency diseases with the nutritional factor whose absence provoked these conditions:

_____ 1.   childhood blindness   a. protein

_____ 2.   marasmus   b. fiber

_____ 3.   anemia   c. vitamin A

_____ 4.   kwashiorkor   d. vitamin B1 (thiamine)

_____ 5.   mental retardation   e. vitamin C

_____ 6.   pellagra   f. vitamin D

_____ 7.   scurvy   g. vitamin E

_____ 8.   rickets   h. niacin

_____ 9.   beri-beri   i. iodine

                                   j. iron

                                   k. overall calorie/protein shortage

C. True/False. If statement is false, revise it below in the space provided to make a correct statement; focus your response on the words in bold.

_____ 1. As incomes rise, food demand increases because more affluent people eat **larger quantities of food.**

_____ 2. It is estimated that approximately **a billion** people in the world today are undernourished.

_____ 3. Within families in poor societies, **adolescent boys** are the most likely to suffer from malnutrition.

_____ 4. **Overpopulation** is the major cause of chronic hunger problems in the developing world.

_____ 5. In societies where hunger is widespread, **the rate of malnutrition among children and women is much higher than it is among men.**

_____ 6. Malnutrition is most harmful when it occurs among **children under 5.**

_____ 7. The damaging effects of childhood malnutrition **are reversible** if the child receives an adequate diet when he/she becomes older.

_____ 8. Malnourished women are likely to **give birth to underweight babies and to produce poor quality breast milk.**

_____ 9. **Marasmus** is responsible for more childhood deaths in developing countries than any other single cause.

_____ 10. The most common nutritional deficiency disease worldwide is **kwashiorkor.**

_____ 11. A swollen belly, discoloration of the hair and skin, and stunted physical development are all classic symptoms of **overall protein/calorie deprivation.**

_____ 12. The world's single most important cause of preventable brain damage and mental retardation is **Vitamin A** deficiency.

_____ 13. Aquaculture offers **greater hope** for increasing the world's fish harvest than does intensifying efforts in ocean fishing.

_____ 14. World livestock production, which rose steadily from 1950–1990, has subsequently leveled off because of **falling market demand for meat.**

Name _____

_____ 15. **Anemia** is a leading cause of high female mortality rates and problem pregnancies in many poor countries.

_____ 16. Aquaculture supplies almost all of the **tuna fish** found in American supermarkets.

_____ 17. Biotechnology can **help reduce farmers' reliance on chemical fertilizers and pesticides and may make it possible to cultivate lands currently too dry or too saline for farming**.

_____ 18. Among species commonly raised to supply animal protein for human consumption, **fish** are the most efficient energy converters, requiring just 2–3 pounds of feed to gain one pound of flesh.

_____ 19. In **sub-Saharan Africa,** grain production has remained stagnant at about one ton/ hectare since the early 1960s.

_____ 20. Significant increases in agricultural production achieved by technological breakthroughs such as the "miracle grains" or genetically modified crop and livestock varieties will **ensure that all the world's people enjoy an adequate diet.**

D. Short Essays:

1. What is meant by the "Green Revolution"? How successful has it been to date in eradicating world hunger? What are its chances of doing so in the years ahead? Are GMOs likely to have an equivalent impact in the near future?

2. Explain why the United States is experiencing an obesity epidemic. What health problems does excessive weight gain cause and what policy actions could be taken to reverse current trends?

3. What are some of the reasons advanced in favor of becoming a "locavore"? To what extent can eating locally reduce one's carbon footprint? Can you suggest another approach that would be more effective?

••••••• 5 •••••••

Impacts of Growth on Ecosystems

A. Fill-in-the-Blank:

_____ 1. What term has been used to describe people who are forced to leave their homeland due to calamities such as soil erosion, deforestation, or desertification?

_____ 2. On a worldwide basis, what activity is the most significant cause of land degradation?

_____ 3. What is the term used to describe the amount of sustainable soil loss that can be experienced without undermining long-term agricultural productivity—the point at which soil losses due to erosion are no greater than the rate of soil formation?

_____ 4. What is the main strategy promoted by the Natural Resources Conservation Service for reducing present rates of soil erosion?

_____ 5. What is the single largest cause of deforestation?

_____ 6. Where is the pace of deforestation causing the greatest concern?

_____ 7. What is today's most serious "energy crisis" for the majority of the developing world's poor people?

_____ 8. In which region of the world has forest loss due to commercial lumbering been most extensive?

_____ 9. What is the leading cause of deforestation in Central America and in Brazil's Amazon basin?

_____ 10. Approximately what percentage of America's original wetlands acreage has been lost to development?

_____ 11. Which of the 50 states has the largest expanse of wetlands habitat?

_____ 12. What is the greatest threat to biodiversity in central and western Africa?

_____ 13. Give an example of a species currently threatened with extinction due to overhunting.

_____ 14. What is the acronym for the international treaty that regulates trade in specified animal and plant products?

_____ 15. Give an example of an exotic species that has severely disrupted the ecology of many U.S. waterways and caused billions of dollars worth of damage.

_____ 16. Give an example of a species endangered by exposure to toxic chemical pollutants.

_____ 17. How did Asian longhorned beetles enter the U.S.?

_____ 18. Name a species recently taken off the "endangered" or "threatened" list.

_____ 19. Cite the most common method by which exotic species are now entering the United States.

_____ 20. Which U.S. state has the highest rate of bird and plant extinctions?

_____ 21. Name a species thought to have been driven to extinction by global warming.

_____ 22. What is the single greatest threat to biodiversity today?

_____ 23. Give an example of a successful community-based conservation effort.

_____ 24. How many U.S. plant and animal species are currently listed as "endangered" or "threatened"?

_____ 25. What is an alternative to the traditional case-by-case approach to protecting species—an innovative way of balancing pressures for economic growth with the need to preserve habitat?

B. Short-Answer Questions:

1. Give some examples of current ecologic situations that are forcing large numbers of people to become "environmental refugees."

2. a) From a soil fertility standpoint, why is it important that current rates of soil erosion be reduced?

   b) Why have crop yields in the U.S. not yet declined in spite of significant soil loss?

   c) How has the Conservation Reserve Program promoted efforts to reduce soil loss in the U.S.?

3. Explain how climate change is likely to impact the long-term survival of coral reefs.

4. What provisions of the Endangered Species Act have had the greatest impact in protecting ecosystems from human pressures?

C. Essay:

Discuss the major forces contributing to deforestation in the tropics and explain why these forces will be so difficult to control. Explain the consequences of deforestation in terms of the ecological and social problems looming on the horizon as the world's forests vanish.

D. Activity:

Visit a local coffeehouse and inquire whether they carry eco-certified coffee. If not, ask whether they would consider doing so.

Name _____

· · · · · · · *6* · · · · · · ·

Environmental Disease

A. Give the term which best fits each of the following definitions:

_____ 1. a substance that causes birth defects

_____ 2. any change in the genetic make-up of a cell

_____ 3. a section along a chromosome, consisting of approximately 1500 base pairs, responsible for the production of a particular protein

_____ 4. a mutation at the molecular level within a gene

_____ 5. a substance that can induce a mutation

_____ 6. threadlike structures within the nucleus of a cell that can be observed under a microscope at the time of cell division

_____ 7. gross structural changes in a chromosome usually caused by loss, addition, or reversal of chromosome parts

_____ 8. a substance that can cause cancer

_____ 9. an irreversible change in the genetic material caused by a brief interaction with a cancer-causing substance

_____ 10. situation in which the interaction of two or more substances produces an effect greater than the sum of their independent effects

_____ 11. the time between the initial exposure of a cell to a cancer-causing substance and the subsequent development of a malignancy

_____ 12. substance that, after prolonged contact, can cause a cell which was previously exposed to a cancer-causing agent to commence malignant growth

_____ 13. genes that give instructions for cells to begin dividing

_____ 14. mutant genes that cause cells to divide endlessly when they should not

_____ 15. genes that act to halt uncontrolled multiplication of cells

B. Fill-in-the-Blank:

_____ 1. What is the hereditary material sometimes referred to as the "Master Molecule"?

a) _____ 2. What are the two main functions of this substance that make it so important to the life of a cell?

b) _____

_____ 3. What is the normal human chromosome number?

_____ 4. Name a human ailment caused by the presence of one additional chromosome per cell.

_____ 5. What is the configuration of the DNA molecule that accounts for its unique characteristics?

_____ 6. Name a human disease caused by a single point mutation.

_____ 7. Give an example of a substance that can act as a mutagen, a teratogen, and a carcinogen.

_____ 8. Name a microbial disease caused by a so-called "newly emerging" pathogen.

a) _____ 9. a) During which weeks of fetal development is vulnerability to teratogenic agents greatest?

b) _____ b) Why is this particular period most critical?

_____ 10. Name an infectious disease against which all women should be immunized prior to reaching childbearing age.

_____ 11. What type of birth defect was caused by prenatal exposure to thalidomide?

_____ 12. What teratogenic drug, taken to prevent miscarriage, caused serious health problems that weren't manifested until victims exposed *in utero* reached young adulthood?

_____ 13. What teratogen is responsible for by far the largest number of birth abnormalities and miscarriages?

_____ 14. Is there a threshold level for exposure to a teratogenic agent?

_____ 15. Neural tube defects could largely be prevented if pregnant women receive adequate amounts of what dietary supplement?

_____ 16. What percentage of deaths in industrialized nations today are caused by some form of cancer?

Name _____

_____ 17. Currently, what is the situation in the U.S. regarding the incidence rate of cancer in general?

_____ 18. What type of cancer kills the most people each year?

_____ 19. Why have mortality rates for uterine cancer declined drastically in recent decades?

_____ 20. What common characteristic is shared by the various diseases collectively called "cancer"?

a) _____ 21. Cite two reasons to justify the standard procedure of testing for carcinogenicity by administering very large doses to laboratory animals.

b) _____

_____ 22. Name a type of cancer associated with a virus infection.

_____ 23. Give an example of a synergistic relationship regarding cancer risk.

a) _____ 24. a) Name a naturally occurring carcinogen found in certain foods.

b) _____   b) Give an example of a food sometimes contaminated with this carcinogen.

a) _____ 25. a) Name an anti-carcinogen found in certain foods.

b) _____   b) Give an example of a food containing this substance.

_____ 26. Name a kind of cancer for which a genetic predisposition has been established.

_____ 27. What single carcinogenic agent is responsible for over 30% of all U.S. cancer deaths?

_____ 28. What dietary factors are most closely correlated with an enhanced risk of colon and prostate cancer?

_____ 29. More than half of all human cancers studied have been shown to contain a mutant form of what gene?

_____ 30. What does the Hazard Communication Standard, promulgated by OSHA in 1983, require that employers do to enhance worker health and safety?

C. Essay:

Recent surveys indicate that teenage girls smoke as much as teenage boys. From the standpoint of both personal and reproductive health, discuss why this fact is particularly unfortunate. Why do you think that young women in particular are adopting a habit widely acknowledged as harmful? Can you suggest effective approaches for reversing this trend?

D. Activity:

In recent years the emphasis on cancer prevention strategies has focused increasingly on changes in personal life-style. Keeping in mind the established factors associated with cancer causation, make a list of your own personal habits and activities that might enhance your risk of someday developing a malignancy. To what extent are you able and/or willing to make changes in your life to reduce such risks?

· · · · · · · · 7 · · · · · · · ·

Toxic Substances

A. Name a toxic substance discussed in Chapter 7 that has been associated with the following diseases or conditions:

_____   1. lung cancer

_____   2. gout

_____   3. fetal brain damage

_____   4. learning disabilities

_____   5. chloracne

_____   6. mesothelioma

_____   7. anemia

_____   8. Minamata Disease

_____   9. disruption of hormonal system

_____   10. Mad Hatters' Disease

B. Indicate the primary route of entry into the human body for each of the following toxic substances, using the following representative symbols:

A = inhalation   (Note: some items may have more than one correct answer)
B = ingestion
C = skin absorption

_____ 1. PCBs
_____ 2. dioxin
_____ 3. asbestos
_____ 4. lead
_____ 5. inorganic mercury
_____ 6. methyl mercury

C. True/False. If statement is false, revise it below in the space provided to make a correct statement; focus your response on the words in bold.

_____ 1. **PCBs** are very useful synthetic organic chemicals that have been used in a wide range of industrial products.

_____ 2. In spite of the fact that PCBs were developed strictly for industrial use, **they have become very widespread throughout the natural environment.**

_____ 3. Elevated levels of **mercury** have been found in farmed salmon due to contamination of their feed with this toxic substance.

_____ 4. When taken into living organisms, PCBs accumulate in the **bones.**

_____ 5. The most common adverse health effect associated with PCB exposure is **liver cancer.**

_____ 6. The food most directly associated with increasing human body levels of PCBs is **freshwater fish.**

_____ 7. There is no convincing evidence that PCBs cause any **chronic** health problems in humans.

_____ 8. TCDD (dioxin) **has been manufactured for use in hundreds of valuable commercial products.**

_____ 9. Dioxin is a **very stable chemical,** persisting in soils for many years after deposition.

_____ 10. Dioxin's reputation as an extremely toxic chemical is due to the fact that **hamsters** are quickly killed by very minute doses of TCDD.

_____ 11. Bisphenol A has been shown to induce **liver cancer** in humans even at low levels of exposure.

_____ 12. Asbestosis develops **only after years of exposure to high concentrations of asbestos fibers.**

_____ 13. Ingesting asbestos with drinking water, as opposed to inhaling asbestos fibers, does **not** appear to increase the risk of asbestos-related disease.

_____ 14. **Mesothelioma** is currently the leading cause of asbestos-related death in the U.S.

_____ 15. Only **friable** asbestos presents serious health concerns in public buildings.

_____ 16. The 1986 Asbestos Hazard Emergency Response Act not only requires schools to inspect for the presence of asbestos but also **to carry out an abatement plan if asbestos-containing materials are found.**

_____ 17. **Encapsulation** is the most commonly chosen asbestos abatement option.

_____ 18. The recommended method for disposal of asbestos wastes following an abatement project is **burial in a sanitary landfill.**

_____ 19. **Carrots, beets, and potatoes** are more likely to be contaminated with lead than are spinach and lettuce.

_____ 20. Lead-base housepaint **is** still causing lead-poisoning cases among children.

_____ 21. Lead that is **inhaled** poses less risk to adults than does lead that is ingested, because most of it is quickly exhaled.

_____ 22. Occupational exposure to mercury fumes is widespread among **dentists and dental hygienists.**

_____ 23. Inorganic forms of mercury are **more** toxic to humans than are organic mercury compounds such as methyl mercury.

_____ 24. **Lung damage,** especially lung cancer, is the major problem experienced by those who inhale mercury vapors.

_____ 25. **Mercury** is an example of a toxic substance that bioaccumulates as it moves up the food chain.

D. Fill-in-the-Blank:

_____ 1. A chemical that can damage health when exposure to repeated low doses occurs over an extended time period can be said to exhibit (____?____) toxicity.

_____ 2. What is the term used to describe the acute toxicity of a chemical?

_____ 3. On a dose-response curve, what is the term used to indicate the point at which the previously horizontal line begins to curve upward?

_____ 4. In assessing health risk, how do investigators typically determine whether or not the substance in question poses a threat to humans?

_____ 5. For purposes of regulation, what assumption regarding carcinogens currently prevails for assessing cancer risk?

_____ 6. What is the least reliable and most problematic step in the risk assessment process?

_____ 7. Name a toxic substance discussed in this chapter for which no level of exposure can be considered safe.

_____ 8. What is regarded as the most important environmental health problem affecting American children?

a) _____ 9. Cigarette smoking significantly enhances the risk of which two asbestos-related diseases?

b) _____

_____ 10. Name a source of human exposure to bisphenol-A.

a) _____ 11. Name two ways in which lead is currently entering the environment.

b) _____

_____ 12. Cite one reason why human exposure to lead has declined in recent years.

a) _____ 13. Give two examples of how PCBs have escaped from the industrial environment to become the most widespread of all environmental contaminants.

b) _____

_____ 14. What is the single most frequent cause of childhood lead poisoning?

_____ 15. What constitutes the largest source of dioxin entering the environment at present?

_____ 16. What ailment is considered a "marker disease" for asbestos exposure due to the fact that asbestos is the only known cause of this illness?

_____ 17. What specific public health concern was the main factor in EPA's decision to phase out the use of leaded gasoline?

_____ 18. What painful treatment method is prescribed for severe lead-poisoning cases?

_____ 19. What policy action did the EPA take in 1993 in order to protect waterfowl from lead poisoning?

_____ 20. Where in the body does dioxin accumulate?

_____ 21. Lead poisoning in adults due to occupational exposure is most common among those engaged in what kind of work?

_____ 22. The 1976 Toxic Substances Control Act specifically banned the production and use of what substance?

_____ 23. In modern times, which of the toxic substances discussed in this chapter has been responsible for the largest incidence of deaths and disabling disease?

_____ 24. What are the two main health concerns underlying government asbestos abatement mandates?

_____ 25. If a previously healthy individual suddenly began complaining of severe stomach pains, vomiting, and constant fatigue, appeared unusually irritable and quarrelsome, and lost his/her appetite, an alert observer might suspect the possibility of poisoning with what toxic substance?

· · · · · · · *8* · · · · · · ·

Pests and Pesticides

A. **Match the following pest-borne diseases with the appropriate vector:**
(Note: some answers may be used more than once)

_____ 1. Lyme disease   a. mosquitoes

_____ 2. cholera   b. houseflies

_____ 3. encephalitis   c. body lice

_____ 4. typhus fever   d. head lice

_____ 5. typhoid fever   e. rat fleas

_____ 6. yellow fever   f. cat fleas

_____ 7. Rocky Mt. spotted fever   g. mites

_____ 8. dengue fever   h. American dog tick

_____ 9. bubonic plague   i. black-legged tick

_____ 10. malaria   j. bedbug

_____ 11. dysentery   k. rodents

_____ 12. scabies   l. brown recluse spider

_____ 13. West Nile virus

Name _____

B. Fill-in-the-Blank:

_____ 1. Which pest-borne disease kills the most people each year?

_____ 2. What recently introduced mosquito-borne disease has spread across the United States, causing numerous fatalities?

a) _____ 3. a) What were the major insecticides used in the U.S. until the end of World War II?

b) _____ b) How did they differ from the newer pesticides introduced after the war?

_____ 4. Name an insect against which a stomach poison would be ineffective.

_____ 5. What is the route of entry of a contact poison (i.e. how does it kill the target pest)?

_____ 6. What are herbicides intended to kill?

a) _____ 7. Give examples of (a) a selective and (b) a nonselective herbicide.

b) _____

_____ 8. For what accomplishment did Paul Muller win the 1948 Nobel Prize in Physiology and Medicine?

_____ 9. What was the name of the chemical defoliant used by the U.S. military during the Vietnam War?

_____ 10. What constituent of this pesticide (#9) is blamed for the alleged health damage associated with its use?

_____ 11. When did the insecticide DDT first come into widespread commercial use?

_____ 12. What book by Rachel Carson, published in 1962, first alerted the general public to the problems posed by pesticides?

_____ 13. Name a mosquito repellent advocated by EPA as both safe and effective for people of all ages.

_____ 14. What is the term used to describe the process by which toxic substances that are present in only minute amounts in the general environment become more and more concentrated as they move up the food chain?

_____ 15. Which group of synthetic organic insecticides has caused serious environmental problems because of their tendency to concentrate in this manner (in reference to preceding question)?

_____ 16. Which group of contact poisons is most acutely toxic to the applicator and hence is the cause of most human pesticide poisonings?

83

_____   17. What serious health problem often affects children living in cockroach-infested residences?

_____   18. Precisely what does the statement "EPA-Registered" mean when it appears on the label of a pesticidal product?

_____   19. Name a spider whose bite leaves a large, ugly scar.

_____   20. What exotic pest entered the U.S. in shipments of old tire casings and subsequently spread throughout large areas of the country?

_____   21. What serious mosquito-borne disease is spreading northward from the tropics as global temperatures gradually rise?

_____   22. What is the first and most obvious symptom of Lyme disease?

a)_____   23. How are the second and third stages of Lyme disease manifested?

b)_____

_____   24. What pest can enter homes and cause severe allergic reactions or dermatitis when sparrows or starlings are allowed to nest on eaves or windowsills?

a)_____   25. a) What type of chemical rodenticides are available to the general public?

b)_____   b) Why are these considered relatively safe to use?

Name _____

C. Discussion Question:

a) As society strives to reduce its reliance on chemical pesticides, describe some practical and effective IPM approaches that you, as a concerned citizen, could pursue in trying to control insects, weeds, and other pests in your own yard and garden.

b) Cite several of the human health and environmental problems the IPM approach to pest control aims to avoid.

D. Short Discussion Questions:

1. Explain why some public health officials in tropical countries advocate the continued use of DDT for malaria control. What are some of the other strategies employed in the ongoing struggle to combat this disease?

2. Cite some reasons why informed consumers have reason to be skeptical about the safety of using many of the pesticides currently on the market.

E. Activity:

Carry out a survey, both indoors and around the outside perimeter of the house, apartment building, or dormitory in which you are living, to determine whether your residence has any kind of pest infestation problem (e.g., rodents, cockroaches, bats, stored food pests, flies, mosquitoes, etc.). Bearing in mind the importance of good housekeeping practices to minimize food, water, and harborage, as well as structural features that "build pests out," list as many potential or actual problem areas as you can find and indicate how principles of good sanitation could be applied to eliminate or prevent infestations.

· · · · · · · · *9* · · · · · · · ·

Food Quality

A. Explain the distinction between the following food quality problems and describe the relative degree of risk each poses to the health of the modern American consumer:

1. *adulterants*

2. *contaminants*

3. *additives*

4. *foodborne disease*

B. Fill-in-the-Blank:

_____ 1. Food Defect Action Levels have been set by the federal government to regulate what kind of food quality problem?

_____ 2. What agency of the federal government regulates food additives and contaminants?

_____ 3. What approach has the government taken for regulating pesticide levels on agricultural products?

_____ 4. What does the Delaney Clause prohibit?

_____ 5. Give an example of a useful food additive that presents no health threat to the majority of consumers but which can provoke a serious allergic reaction among a sizeable minority.

a) _____ 6. a) Name a substance that has been taken off the list of approved food additives.

b) _____ b) Why was it removed?

_____ 7. What previously neglected issue related to children's health was addressed as part of the 1996 Food Quality Protection Act?

_____ 8. What food quality problem is likely to be greater with imported foods than with U.S.-grown products?

_____ 9. What controversial food product is the subject of an acrimonious food safety debate between the U.S. and the European Union?

_____ 10. What plant is responsible for more fatal poisonings due to misidentification than any other species?

_____ 11. Ciguatoxin is a poison found in _____.

_____ 12. Consumption of tuna fish that aren't properly chilled after catching may result in a type of food poisoning called _____, caused by ingestion of a bacterial toxin.

_____ 13. Shellfish sanitation and inspection programs are rigorously implemented by the federal government to forestall outbreaks of _____, a form of food poisoning caused when clams or oysters become contaminated with an algal toxin.

_____ 14. What type of food quality problem has become increasingly common among lovers of sushi and ceviche?

_____ 15. What food is the leading cause of *Campylobacter* food poisoning?

_____ 16. Contamination with what substance has been identified as the source of *E. coli 0157:H7* organisms on foods as diverse as raw beef and alfalfa sprouts?

_____ 17. For what bacterial foodborne disease do symptoms appear most rapidly after eating the contaminated food?

_____ 18. What chronic health problem may result as a consequence of a salmonellosis infection?

_____ 19. What foodborne disease has the highest mortality rate?

_____ 20. Which foodborne disease organism can be transmitted by sneeze droplets or pus coming into contact with food?

_____ 21. What precautions should be followed by home canners to prevent the threat of botulism?

a) _____ 22. a) Name a foodborne disease whose causative agent, unlike most foodborne disease pathogens, multiplies rapidly at low temperatures.

b) _____ b) For which segment of the population is this disease particularly dangerous?

_____ 23. What effect does freezing food have in terms of preventing bacterial foodborne disease?

_____ 24. What is the most toxic substance known?

_____ 25. What is the "Danger Zone" in terms of the temperature range that will support the multiplication of food poisoning bacteria?

_____ 26. What is the most frequent lapse in time-temperature control leading to outbreaks of foodborne illness?

_____ 27. What is the term used to describe the transmission of foodborne pathogens from one food item to another via equipment or workers' hands?

_____ 28. It is now recognized that even whole, uncracked eggs, formerly thought to be safe, can be contaminated with what foodborne disease organism?

a) _____ 29. For which two bacterial foodborne diseases is the infectious dose very low?

b) _____

_____ 30. What is the most frequent cause for outbreaks of viral foodborne diseases?

C. Short Discussion Questions:

1. Explain the rationale behind the federal government's approach to regulating contaminants in food.

2. Why do most food safety experts deplore the continued subtherapeutic use of antibiotics in livestock feed and trough water? What evidence suggests their fears are well-founded?

3. a) Give examples of "potentially hazardous foods"—those most frequently associated with outbreaks of bacterial foodborne disease.

   b) What are some foods that seldom cause such problems? Why?

4. Distinguish between food spoilage and foodborne disease, explaining why the common practice of sniffing leftovers prior to eating them is no guarantee of food safety.

5. Why is time-temperature control the key to preventing food poisoning outbreaks?

6. List the points you would raise in an effort to convince a friend that irradiated food is safe to eat.

D. Activity:

Observe food preparation activities in a home kitchen, restaurant, school cafeteria, or any other food service area to which you have access. Make a list of situations or procedures that could potentially lead to foodborne disease outbreaks. Take special note of such factors as personal hygiene among food handlers, frequency of hand washing, cleaning of knives and cutting boards after each use, food temperatures, etc.

Summarize your observations and indicate whether perceived violations of good food sanitation practices were a result of ignorance, carelessness, or lack of adequate facilities. What practical suggestions could you offer to improve food-handling procedures?

·········10·········

Radiation

A. True/False. If statement is false, revise it below in the space provided to make a correct statement; focus your response on the words in bold.

_____ 1. The existence of ionizing radiation in the form of "x-rays" was discovered by **Marie Curie.**

_____ 2. Because of its ability to destroy chemical bonds, ionizing radiation is **more damaging** to living organisms than is non-ionizing radiation.

_____ 3. **Gamma rays** are the most energetic but least penetrating form of ionizing radiation.

_____ 4. **Alpha particles** present a health threat only when they are taken internally through inhalation or ingestion or when an open wound permits contact with delicate internal tissues.

_____ 5. Exposure to cosmic rays has **no adverse human health impact.**

_____ 6. **Beta radiation** can pass through the skin but is more dangerous when ingested with food or water.

_____ 7. **Beta radiation and x-rays** have basically the same characteristics.

_____ 8. For the average American, **medical or dental x-rays** represent the largest single source of exposure to ionizing radiation.

_____ 9. **All radiation exposure is cumulative.**

_____ 10. Next to medical uses of radiation, **nuclear weapons fallout** is the most significant source of public exposure to human-made radiation.

_____ 11. Currently most people receive approximately **half their annual radiation exposure from natural sources, half from human-made sources.**

_____ 12. Among consumer products, the most significant source of radiation exposure is **cigarettes.**

_____ 13. People living in the vicinity of nuclear power plants receive **minimal** radiation exposure from these facilities.

_____ 14. Reinterpretation of data regarding radiation exposure of Japanese survivors at Hiroshima suggests that current federal radiation safety standards are **overly protective** in their attempt to prevent cancer and genetic defects.

_____ 15. The half-life of a radioactive substance represents **the length of time it poses a threat to living organisms.**

_____ 16. A given amount of radiation will be **less** harmful to insects than to humans.

_____ 17. People who survive high-level exposure to radiation are **still at much higher risk than the general public** of subsequently developing cancer or producing defective offspring.

_____ 18. The most dangerous time for fetal exposure to ionizing radiation is **the period shortly before birth.**

_____ 19. The piles of radioactive "tailings" located near uranium mills represent the **greatest source of public exposure to ionizing radiation related to nuclear power production.**

_____ 20. There are currently **two** nuclear fuel reprocessing facilities operating in the U.S.

_____ 21. Under the provisions of the 1980 Low-Level Radioactive Waste Policy Act, the **federal** government has the authority to regulate and manage the disposal of all U.S. low-level radioactive wastes.

_____ 22. Each year more new cases of **skin cancer** are diagnosed than of any other type of cancer.

_____ 23. **Malignant melanoma** is the most common form of skin cancer in the U.S.

_____ 24. According to dermatologists, sunscreens must have a minimum **SPF of 8** to prevent skin damage.

_____ 25. Body parts that are **moist and that have poor circulation—e.g. eyes, G-I tract, testes, etc.—**are those most likely to be damaged by microwaves.

_____ 26. The most challenging radioactive waste management problems are presented by those radioactive elements with **extremely long half-lives.**

_____ 27. With the possible exception of carcinogens, the health damage caused by a given quantity of radiation will be less if **exposure occurs over an extended time period as opposed to being delivered all at once.**

_____ 28. **Leukemia** has been the most common health effect responsible for increased morbidity and mortality among those living near the Chernobyl nuclear power plant at the time of the 1986 accident.

_____ 29. In order to reduce greenhouse gas emissions, several countries in **western Europe** are committed to increasing their reliance on nuclear power for meeting growing energy demands.

_____ 30. Most sunscreens provide protection against **UVB only.**

B. Fill-in-the-Blank:

_____ 1. What is the unit for measuring radiation damage in humans?

_____ 2. What amount of radiation exposure constitutes high-level exposure?

_____ 3. What range of health effects could high-level radiation exposure entail?

_____ 4. What are the primary health concerns regarding low-level radiation exposure?

_____ 5. What is the worst type of accident that could occur at a nuclear power plant?

_____ 6. What would cause most of the casualties if a "dirty bomb" were detonated in a U.S. city?

a) _____ 7. What two fissionable materials are retrieved from spent nuclear fuel rods during fuel reprocessing?

b) _____

_____ 8. Fear of what possible threat led President Carter to impose a moratorium on reprocessing of commercial nuclear fuel?

_____ 9. How are high-level radioactive wastes from commercial nuclear power plants currently being managed?

_____ 10. What health problems have been conclusively linked with exposure to depleted uranium munitions?

_____ 11. What sorts of radioactive waste are destined for disposal at the Waste Isolation Pilot Plant (WIPP) in New Mexico?

_____ 12. Give an example of low-level radioactive waste.

a) _____ 13. Name two ways in which low-level radioactive wastes differ from high-level wastes.

b) _____

_____ 14. What is the biological effect of ultraviolet radiation?

_____ 15. What is the major health problem associated with ultraviolet light?

_____ 16. Name one problem caused by UVB radiation that does not occur with UVA exposure.

_____ 17. What impact do microwaves have on absorbing materials?

_____ 18. What region of the world is considered by experts to be the likeliest source for terrorists to obtain a "loose nuke"?

_____ 19. What ailment in young or middle-aged adults is associated with a severe blistering sunburn during childhood or adolescence?

_____ 20. What form of cancer is most frequently associated with exposure to ionizing radiation?

_____ 21. Where on the body do basal cell carcinomas most commonly occur?

_____ 22. What is likely to happen if a person taking antibiotics, antihistamines, or a number of other drugs visits a tanning parlor or sunbathes outdoors?

a) _____ 23. Name two potential problems that are just as likely to occur among patrons of tanning parlors as they are among sunbathers on a beach.

b) _____

_____ 24. What is the current position of the National Academy of Sciences regarding the human health impact of exposure to electromagnetic fields (EMFs)?

C. Essay:

Are you in favor of meeting future U.S. energy needs through increased reliance on nuclear power? Defend your position on this important public policy question.

Name _____

D. Activity:

Contact the office in charge of environmental health and safety on your campus and inquire whether radioactive wastes are generated at your college or university. If so, ask:

• What departments or offices are the sources of such materials?

• What types of radioactive wastes do they generate?

• How are such wastes managed on campus?

• Where are they ultimately sent for disposal?

• What does your institution spend each year for radioactive waste management?

• Do the authorities in charge of campus radwaste management anticipate future problems in finding a disposal site able and willing to receive such wastes?

• • • • • • • • 1 1 • • • • • • • •

The Atmosphere

A. Fill-in-the-Blank:

_____ 1. What gas do scientists currently believe was the major component of the primitive Earth's atmosphere?

_____ 2. What change was responsible for making the modern Earth's atmosphere one rich in oxygen?

_____ 3. On what basis is the atmosphere divided into its various regions?

_____ 4. Which region of the atmosphere is nearest to the earth's surface?

_____ 5. In which atmospheric region does the ozone layer occur?

_____ 6. The major portion of which form of solar radiation is absorbed as it passes through the atmosphere, with only a tiny fraction of the original amount reaching the surface of the earth?

_____ 7. What form of solar radiation is absorbed by both carbon dioxide and water vapor?

_____ 8. Of the major atmospheric gases, which is the only one whose concentration has been increasing during the past century?

a) _____ 9. In reference to the preceding question, what two factors are largely responsible for this increase?

b) _____

_____ 10. What consequence of this increase is feared by atmospheric scientists?

_____ 11. What pollutant represents a serious threat to the integrity of the ozone layer?

_____ 12. What would be the human health consequences of ozone layer destruction?

_____ 13. Over which region of the world has ozone loss been most significant?

_____ 14. What international treaty went into effect in 1989, aimed at mustering worldwide efforts to protect the ozone layer?

_____ 15. What is the major action called for by this treaty?

_____ 16. What country is the largest emitter of CO_2 to the atmosphere?

_____ 17. What new approach is being proposed to continue burning coal without further endangering the atmosphere?

a) _____ 18. Give two examples of "positive feedbacks" that could magnify the rise of temperature associated with global warming.

b) _____

_____ 19. Above what level of temperature increase do most scientists agree the consequences will be catastrophic?

_____ 20. According to some scientists, on which pollutant should control efforts be focused immediately as the quickest, easiest way to mitigate climate change?

Name _____

B. Short Discussion Questions:

1. What is meant by the "Greenhouse Effect"? What are the problems that might accompany a global warming trend?

2. What role do trace gases such as CFCs and methane play in relation to the Greenhouse Effect?

3. Cite several pieces of recently acquired scientific evidence supporting those who believe global warming has already begun. What additional impacts are likely to become apparent during your lifetime?

C. Essay:

Many people, including supposedly knowledgeable media personalities, confuse the issues of ozone layer depletion and global warming. Using the chart below, compare and contrast these two serious, but different, atmospheric problems.

	Ozone Layer Depletion	Global Warming
Major cause of problem		
Type of solar radiation absorbed		
Potential human health impact		
Environmental consequences		
International treaty for resolving issue		
Solution to problem		
Is effective action being taken?		

D. Activity:

Contact your congressional representative and ask what policy actions, if any, he or she would support to avert global climate change. In your opinion, what political or economic realities influence his or her position on this issue? Has your state government passed legislation to deal with climate change?

12

Clean Energy Alternatives

A. Fill-in-the-blank:

_____ 1. What percentage of world energy use currently is derived from fossil fuels?

_____ 2. Major new reserves of what fossil fuel have recently been discovered in the United States?

_____ 3. What do energy experts regard as the most promising option for reducing dependence on fossil fuels in the near-term?

_____ 4. Putting on a sweater instead of turning up the heat on a cold winter day represents an example of energy _____.

_____ 5. What U.S. government program is intended to aid consumers in choosing energy-efficient appliances and computers?

_____ 6. Name the voluntary certification system for identifying "green" buildings.

_____ 7. What federal fuel efficiency standard must the U.S. motor vehicle fleet meet by 2016?

_____ 8. What renewable energy source currently has the fastest growth rate?

_____ 9. Name one factor restricting the growth of nuclear power.

_____ 10. Name one of the three U.S. states with the highest potential for wind electricity generation.

_____ 11. What is the primary purpose for which solar thermal collectors are currently being used?

_____ 12. What is the main factor limiting the siting of large concentrating solar power (CSP) facilities in the U.S.?

_____ 13. What country depends on geothermal power for more than half its total energy demand?

_____ 14. What is the major feedstock for biodiesel fuel in the U.S. at the present time?

_____ 15. What form of renewable fuel is being captured at some sanitary landfills?

_____ 16. What do energy experts say is the single most effective action a concerned individual could take to reduce household energy use?

_____ 17. Name a "third-generation biofuel" of interest to farmers in the midwestern U.S. because it is a winter annual that can be double-cropped with soybeans.

_____ 18. What do a number of renewable energy advocates and utility companies argue is the most serious short- and mid-term obstacle to further development of commercial-scale wind and solar electricity?

_____ 19. What U.S. state leads the nation in the number of homes with rooftop solar PV systems?

_____ 20. Give an example of a type of government incentive offered by some states to encourage homeowners to install solar panels.

B. True/False. If statement is false, revise it below in the space provided to make a correct statement; focus your response on the words in bold.

_____ 1. **Oil** now constitutes the single-largest component of U.S. energy consumption.

_____ 2. Energy **efficiency** involves reducing energy consumption by curtailing certain normal activities.

_____ 3. At present, LED bulbs are most commonly used for **outdoor street and traffic lights.**

_____ 4. **The European Union** has banned the sale of incandescent light bulbs starting in 2012.

_____ 5. Homes **built before 1939** are generally less energy efficient than those constructed during the past decade.

_____ 6. The greatest potential for energy savings in transportation lies in **doubling fuel efficiency standards**.

_____ 7. **Wind power** provides over half the renewable energy utilized commercially for electrical generation at the present time.

_____ 8. **Extremely high construction costs** of new power plants are a major deterrent to the further expansion of nuclear energy.

_____ 9. **China** derives a larger percentage of its electricity from wind power than any other nation.

_____ 10. For power plants utilizing wind energy, **natural gas** provides effective backup power during times when the wind isn't blowing.

_____ 11. The oldest concentrating solar power (CSP) plant operating in the U.S. is located in southern California; a newer facility of similar design is now generating electricity in **Arizona**.

_____ 12. **Home heating** constitutes the single largest use of geothermal energy.

_____ 13. A major benefit of biofuel use over that of gasoline is **lower greenhouse gas emissions**.

_____ 14. **Hydrogen fuel cells** represent the most promising option for "greener" cars in the years ahead.

_____ 15. **Jatropha** is widely regarded as the likeliest major source of biofuels in the future, since it yields up to 100 times the amount of oil as soybeans and grows 20–30 times faster.

C. Short-answer questions:

1. List 3 reasons energy experts cite for transitioning as quickly as possible from gasoline or diesel-fueled vehicles to hybrid, electric, or biofuels-powered automobiles and trucks.

2. Why is natural gas regarded as environmentally preferable to coal as an energy source?

3. List 3 features of the American Recovery and Reinvestment Act of 2009 aimed at enhancing U.S. energy efficiency.

4. Give two examples of actions that could improve energy efficiency.

5. Cite two advantages of compact fluorescent bulbs (CFLs) over standard incandescent light bulbs.

6. What specific action do energy experts regard as the quickest, easiest way of reducing household energy demand?

7. Name 3 advantages LED bulbs have over CFLs.

8. What does U.S. law say regarding the status of incandescent light bulbs by 2020?

9. List 3 things you could do in your home or apartment to save energy while using appliances.

10. From an environmental standpoint, what are two advantages of nuclear power over fossil fuels for generating electricity?

11. What advantage could wind energy bring to farmers in Great Plains states?

12. During periods when the sun isn't shining, how do most buildings with rooftop PV systems get their electricity?

Name _____

13. What is the major limitation on greatly expanding our reliance on tidal and wave power?

14. Why are Renewable Energy Standards (RES) important for encouraging the growth of clean energy technologies?

15. What major advantage does distributed generation (DG) of electrical power have over large centralized power plants?

16. What particular advantage do solar water heaters have for rural households in less-developed countries?

D. Discussion Questions:

1. What role do you think nuclear power should play in meeting the world's energy needs over the next several decades? Why?

2. How serious are the problems posed by wind farms to wildlife? Cite several concerns raised by wind farm opponents and assess their validity.

3. Cite the pros and cons of corn ethanol as an alternative to gasoline. Are there other biofuels that offer greater promise? Explain.

4. Describe how the widespread deployment of "smart grid" technology could boost the potential for household energy savings.

· · · · · · · · · 13 · · · · · · · ·

Air Pollution

A. Indicate which of the criteria air pollutants fits each of the following descriptions:

_____ 1. most difficult to control of all the criteria pollutants

_____ 2. coal-burning facilities and metal smelters are the main sources of this pollutant

_____ 3. the only pollutant gas that is colored

_____ 4. importance of this pollutant has steadily declined as a result of mandated changes in the composition of gasoline

_____ 5. the most abundant pollutant gas in cities

_____ 6. the most visible form of air pollution, since it includes all solid and liquid pollutants

_____ 7. the single most significant precursor of acid precipitation

_____ 8. a second important contributor to acid rain

_____ 9. certain tailpipe emissions from automobiles, along with volatile organic compounds from stationary sources, react in the presence of oxygen and sunshine to form this pollutant gas

_____ 10. cigarette smoke is an important source of this pollutant indoors

_____ 11. use of reformulated gasoline is supposed to lower wintertime concentrations of this criteria air pollutant

_____ 12. approximately half the national emissions of this pollutant come from auto exhausts, the other half from coal-burning power plants

_____ 13. this pollutant is held responsible for billions of dollars worth of crop loss annually, even in regions far removed from major sources of pollutant emissions

_____ 14. short-term exposure to this gas can cause headaches and dizziness, as well as a slowing of mental processes and reaction time; exposure to high concentrations can be fatal

_____ 15. the most serious health effects associated with polluted air are caused by this criteria pollutant

B. True/False. If statement is false, revise it below in the space provided to make a correct statement; focus your response on the words in bold.

_____ 1. The first air quality ordinances in the U.S. were **laws regulating the height of smokestacks.**

_____ 2. **Coal-burning factories** represent the single leading source of air pollution in this country.

_____ 3. The term **"criteria air pollutants"** refers to those pollutants that have been judged most dangerous to health.

_____ 4. "Nonattainment areas" are those which **are in violation of one or more of the primary national ambient air quality standards.**

_____ 5. "Photochemical smog" is the **murky mixture of smoke and fog that readers of mystery novels commonly associate with 19th century London.**

_____ 6. During episodes of unusually severe air pollution, virtually all the human deaths **occurred among people who were already suffering from heart or respiratory disease.**

_____ 7. The 1990 Clean Air Act required the use of reformulated gasoline as **a replacement for tetraethyl lead, a performance-enhancing additive banned a few years earlier.**

_____ 8. **Air pollution and cigarette smoking act synergistically,** a fact that explains why smokers in polluted areas are at greater risk of chronic respiratory problems than are smokers living in nonpolluted areas.

_____ 9. Air quality is **much worse** in eastern Europe and in urban areas of developing countries than it is in the U.S. and western Europe.

_____ 10. Citizens living in polluted industrial areas of the U.S. have **no way of knowing whether they are being exposed to health-threatening levels of hazardous air pollutants.**

_____ 11. In regulating airborne particulates, the EPA has set national standards **only for those particles larger than 100 micrometers,** since these present the greatest threat of respiratory tract blockage.

_____ 12. The 1970 Clean Air Act mandated that the primary air quality standards that the EPA was to establish to safeguard human health were to be set **without regard to pollution control costs.**

_____ 13. U.S. air quality in general is **better** today than it was in 1970 when the Clean Air Act was passed.

_____ 14. Virtually every air pollution "disaster" on record occurred when an **inversion layer** was in place.

_____ 15. Our inability to achieve compliance with all the national ambient air quality standards everywhere in the U.S. is due almost entirely to **coal-fired power plants built prior to implementation of 1970 Clean Air Act regulations.**

_____ 16. An epidemiologic study conducted on schoolchildren in Connecticut revealed that the major source of exposure to air pollutants for these young people was **fumes from pesticides and cleaning supplies inside the school building.**

_____ 17. Brief but intense spikes in concentrations of air pollutants can cause **more severe health problems** among sensitive segments of the population than does chronic exposure to lower levels of air contaminants.

_____ 18. EPA's Clean Air Interstate Rule (CAIR), intended to reduce premature deaths in the eastern U.S. and to improve visibility, is targeted specifically at pollution emissions from **diesel trucks and off-road vehicles.**

_____ 19. Leaded gasoline is now outlawed in **most countries of the world.**

_____ 20. Childhood asthma attacks are more often triggered by **indoor air pollutants than by outdoor air pollutants.**

C. Fill-in-the-Blank:

a) _____   1. Name the three tailpipe emissions controlled by the use of a three-way catalytic converter.

b) _____

c) _____

_____   2. During an atmospheric inversion, is air near the ground warmer or cooler than the air above it?

a) _____   3. Cite two ways in which reformulated gasoline differs from conventional gasoline.

b) _____

_____   4. Which geographical area in the U.S. has the most significant acid rain problem?

_____   5. What pH value is generally considered normal for natural, unpolluted rain?

_____   6. What is the average pH of precipitation today throughout the U.S. east of the Mississippi River?

_____   7. What source of pollutant emissions is the main target of acid rain controls?

_____   8. In what way might acid rain affect human health?

_____   9. What pollution control strategy adopted in the early 1970s to combat localized air quality violations actually worsened the acid rain problem?

_____   10. Under the 1990 Clean Air Act Amendments, what market-based approach to reducing SO_2 emissions was adopted in an effort to combat acid rain?

_____   11. What property of radon gas makes it hazardous to health?

_____   12. What health problem is associated with exposure to radon in homes?

_____   13. What is the source of radon in homes?

_____   14. Where in a home are radon concentrations likely to be highest?

_____   15. At what time of year are radon levels generally the highest?

_____   16. What does the EPA consider the "action level" for initiating radon abatement efforts?

_____   17. What is the most significant indoor source of particulate pollution?

Name _____

a) _____ 18. Gas stoves can emit substantial amounts of which two criteria air pollutants?

b) _____

a) _____ 19. Paradichlorobenzene, a known carcinogen, is the active ingredient in what two common household products?

b) _____

_____ 20. Particleboard, plywood, and wood paneling may emit significant amounts of what common indoor air pollutant?

_____ 21. What transportation control strategy has been adopted by many states in order to meet clean air standards?

_____ 22. What tiny living organism inside homes is a frequent cause of allergic reactions among residents?

_____ 23. What is the most frequent cause of "sick building syndrome"?

_____ 24. What presents the greatest risk of contracting an airborne health problem aboard a commercial jetliner?

a) _____ 25. Cite two ways in which hazardous air pollutants (HAPs) differ from criteria pollutants.

b) _____

_____ 26. What is *Stachybotrys chartarum*?

_____ 27. Name a type of popular motor vehicle that emits significantly more pollutant gases than do standard passenger cars.

_____ 28. Loss of what essential soil nutrient is now suspected as a leading cause of reduced forest productivity in regions adversely affected by acid precipitation?

_____ 29. What source of indoor air pollution does the World Health Organization consider one of the most critical environmental health problems in developing countries?

D. Short-Answer Questions:

1. Explain how high levels of air pollution can influence the frequency of bacterial respiratory diseases such as pneumonia or acute bronchitis.

2. Explain why allowance trading has been such a successful strategy in regulatory efforts to reduce acid rain. How does it work?

3. What procedures should you follow to ensure accurate results if you decide to test your home for radon using a home radon test kit?

4. What environmental conditions promote indoor air quality problems caused by *Stachybotrys chartarum*? If such a problem is discovered, what should residents of the affected dwelling do about it?

E. Activity:

Contact the Emergency Services Disaster Agency (ESDA) in your home county and inquire about the nature of the emergency response plan filed under the requirements of Title III: The Emergency Planning and Community-Right-to-Know Act. What are some of the toxic materials manufactured, stored, used, or transported within your community? What facilities are the main source of these materials? Have any toxic releases been reported? How confident are you of the ability of local officials to deal with a chemical emergency in your community should one ever occur?

· · · · · · · · 14 · · · · · · · ·

Noise Pollution

A. Fill-in-the-Blank:

_____ 1. What is the unit used to measure noise levels?

_____ 2. What is the standard unit used for measuring the frequency of sound?

a) _____ 3. Cite two reasons why noise levels in the U.S. are rising.

b) _____

a) _____ 4. a) What level of noise exposure, if experienced on a regular basis, could lead to permanent impairment of hearing ability?

b) _____   b) Give an example of an everyday activity that generates noise of this magnitude.

_____ 5. What is the term used to describe the rate of vibration of an object—how fast it is moving back and forth?

_____ 6. What term is used to describe the *intensity* of sound—the amount of energy behind a sound wave?

_____ 7. What structures within the inner ear can be damaged by noise, resulting in a loss of hearing?

_____ 8. Why is noise-induced hearing loss irreversible?

_____ 9. What term is used to describe the condition characterized by a ringing or buzzing sound in the head?

_____ 10. What recreational activity is the single greatest cause of nonoccupational noise-induced hearing loss?

B. Short-Answer Questions:

1. What is meant by "temporary threshold shift"? Give an example of how this could occur.

2. To what extent does amplified music present a threat of noise-induced hearing loss?

3. Why do environmental groups oppose the U.S. Navy's efforts to deploy its low-frequency active sonar system throughout extensive areas of the ocean?

4. Give some examples of local ordinances aimed at regulating noise levels in a community. Does your hometown make any effort to control noise?

5. Why have federal and state noise control programs been markedly less successful than other environmental programs? What changes in public attitudes are needed if noise abatement efforts are to be effective?

C. Activity:

Survey 10 people of varying ages and backgrounds, asking them to identify the sources of noise that are most annoying to them. Can you draw any general conclusions from the responses you elicited?

• • • • • • • • 15 • • • • • • • •

Water Resources

A. Draw a word diagram of the hydrologic cycle:

B. Fill-in-the-Blank:

_____ 1. Where does the energy that powers the hydrologic cycle originate?

_____ 2. What percentage of all water on earth consists of fresh water, potentially usable by humans?

_____ 3. How much water is required per person on a daily basis simply to maintain a minimally adequate standard of living?

_____ 4. What region of the U.S. is chronically water-short?

_____ 5. What activity is the nation's single largest consumer of water?

_____ 6. What is the main factor limiting greater reliance on desalination as a means of augmenting water supplies?

_____ 7. From a global perspective, where are conflicts over dwindling water supplies likely to be most acute in the years ahead?

_____ 8. What is the name given to the geologic strata containing groundwater?

_____ 9. What is the term used to describe nonrenewable groundwater reserves formed in the distant past that are no longer being replenished because of geologic and climatic changes?

_____ 10. The upper limit of the Zone of Saturation is referred to as the _____.

_____ 11. What is the major difference in the way in which groundwater flows in comparison with the movement of surface water?

_____ 12. What is the term used to describe the land area where precipitation seeps into the soil and replenishes groundwater reserves?

_____ 13. What is the name of the largest underground water reserve in the world, located in the western U.S., which is being depleted by overpumping?

a) _____ 14. Cite two reasons why it is unlikely that any large new dams will be built in the United States in the foreseeable future.

b) _____

_____ 15. Where is the world's largest dam?

_____ 16. Name one environmental benefit of this project cited by dam proponents.

_____ 17. Name one environmental problem expected as a result of dam construction.

_____ 18. To meet future U.S. water demands, state and municipal leaders are now taking what new approach as an alternative to the supply augmentation projects of past years?

_____ 19. By law, all new or replacement toilets sold in the U.S. must be models using only _____ gallons of water per flush.

_____ 20. What practice is expected to provide the largest source of additional water to meet U.S. needs in the decades ahead?

_____ 21. What is the term used to describe the horticultural practice of choosing plant varieties that don't need supplemental watering?

_____ 22. Where are the largest number of desalination plants currently located?

_____ 23. In what large developing country does "groundwater mining" pose a serious threat to that nation's future harvests?

_____ 24. Who will be the main beneficiaries of China's South-to-North Water Transfer Project?

_____ 25. What do many experts consider the primary cause for overuse and waste of water resources?

C. Short-Answer Questions:

1. Explain how availability and accessibility of safe water supplies can have an impact on human health.

2. Briefly describe how existing water resources in the U.S. are being needlessly wasted and suggest several ways such losses could be reduced.

3. What advantages does groundwater have over surface water as a source of a community's drinking water supply?

4. List potential sources of groundwater contamination and indicate policies that could be adopted to prevent such contamination from occurring.

5. What are some arguments for and against treating water as a commodity to be bought and sold like any other product in the world marketplace?

6. Cite several areas of the world where disputes over water supplies could lead to conflict either between or within countries.

D. Activity:

List ways in which you personally use more water than necessary. What changes in habits or practices could you adopt to use water more efficiently? Do you feel that making such changes would seriously affect your quality of life?

· · · · · · · · · 16 · · · · · · · ·

Water Pollution

A. Explain the meaning of the following terms and indicate their relevance to water quality concerns:

1. Biochemical Oxygen Demand (BOD)

2. eutrophication

3. "point source" of water pollution

4. "nonpoint source" of water pollution

5. indirect discharges

6. pretreatment requirements

7. biosolids

8. SOCs

9. combined sewer overflows

10. hypoxia

B. Fill-in-the-Blank:

_____   1. What type of water contaminants present the greatest health threat to most residents of developing countries?

_____   2. What water pollutants are currently the main focus of concern in industrialized nations?

a) _____   3. What two pollutants are mainly responsible for initiating the process of eutrophication?

b) _____

_____   4. What change occurring in a waterway undergoing eutrophication is the main factor responsible for the loss of fish?

_____   5. What health problems have been confirmed among people who consumed food crops grown on land fertilized with biosolids?

_____   6. Name a type of contaminant often found in sludge from POTWs that receive industrial wastewater discharges.

_____   7. What human activity do scientists blame for the so-called "dead zone" off the coast of Louisiana?

_____   8. What percentage of the American population lives in areas serviced by sewage treatment plants?

_____   9. How is household wastewater managed in most unsewered areas of the country?

_____   10. What minimum level of sewage treatment are all sewage treatment plants in the U.S. required to provide?

a) _____   11. What are the two most common methods of sludge disposal at the present time?

b) _____

a) _____   12. a) Give an example of a method of advanced wastewater treatment.

b) _____   b) What water contaminant is this method designed to remove?

_____   13. The Clean Water Act's Part 503 standards, issued in 1993, specify acceptable management practices for what potential pollutant?

_____   14. What alternative approach to conventional sewage treatment is being adopted by a growing number of communities seeking a less expensive, more environmentally benign method of wastewater treatment?

_____   15. Cite an example of one such method.

_____ 16. What kind of pathogenic organism is responsible for the condition known as "swimmer's itch"?

_____ 17. Name a common source of the pathogens associated with RWIs in swimming pools.

_____ 18. Cite a situation for which bottled water is essential to protect public health.

_____ 19. After what age is the threat of methemoglobinemia no longer a concern?

_____ 20. What dangerous pollutant enters drinking water while passing through the home plumbing system?

a) _____ 21. What simple steps can be taken by householders to avoid consuming excessive amounts of this substance (#20) in their drinking water?

b) _____

_____ 22. Name a group of SOCs, regarded as potential carcinogens, that may be formed at the water treatment plant when chemical disinfectants are added to the raw water supply.

_____ 23. What is the purpose of adding chlorine to sewage treatment plant effluent and to drinking water?

a) _____ 24. Name two waterborne disease organisms that are highly resistant to chlorination.

b) _____

_____ 25. In what country are large numbers of people seriously ill or dying, poisoned by arsenic in their well water?

C. Name some serious waterborne diseases caused by each of the following groups of organisms:

Bacteria

Viruses

Protozoans/Parasitic Worms

D. Short Discussion Questions:

1. Give some examples of nonpoint sources of water pollution. Describe the kinds of pollutants they contribute to waterways and explain why they are proving so much more difficult to control than the point sources.

2. Explain why chlorination of both drinking water and treated effluent from POTWs, once standard procedure, is now generating controversy among environmental health specialists and the public in general. Describe a method for disinfecting water that does not rely on chlorine.

3. How common are recreational water illnesses (RWIs)? Give some examples of health problems associated with swimming pools, hot tubs, or beaches and precautions that can be taken to prevent them.

4. Why do many people argue that bottled water is both bad for the environment and a waste of money?

E. Activity:

Contact your local water treatment plant and obtain information regarding:

• the source of your community's water supply

• what contaminants are present in the raw water supply

• treatment methods used to remove these contaminants

• the existence of any problems in meeting all the mandated MCLs

• methods used by the water treatment plant to inform or educate its customers about water quality problems should they arise

• adequacy of the community water supply for the foreseeable future, given existing growth trends

• adequacy of treatment plant's capacity to meet projected water demand

$\cdots\cdots\cdots 17 \cdots\cdots\cdots$

Solid and Hazardous Wastes

A. Define the following terms and explain their relevance to waste management concerns:

1. leachate

2. tipping fee

3. RCRA Subtitle D

4. "pay-as-you-throw"

5. vermicomposting

6. MRFs

7. brownfields

8. phytoremediation

9. National Priority List (NPL)

10. NIMBY problem

B. True/False. If statement is false, revise it below in the space provided to make a correct statement; focus your response on the words in bold.

_____ 1. Rising volumes of solid waste in the U.S. are primarily related to **an increase in population.**

_____ 2. **Plastics** constitute the single largest portion of the municipal solid waste stream by volume.

_____ 3. Historically, cities have given much greater importance to regular **collection of refuse** than to proper disposal of such materials.

_____ 4. In the U.S. at present it is **illegal to feed garbage to hogs.**

_____ 5. Until more stringent environmental laws were enacted in the 1970s, **incineration** of refuse was the most common method of municipal waste disposal in this country.

_____ 6. The main reason that hundreds of communities are now vigorously involved in municipal recycling programs is because of their concern for saving **resources and energy.**

_____ 7. Open dumps are now **illegal throughout the U.S.**

_____ 8. The major environmental concern with sanitary landfills is the **threat of water pollution** as dissolved materials seep out and contaminate aquifers or surface streams.

_____ 9. **Landfilling** must always be an integral part of any comprehensive waste management plan, since some wastes cannot be disposed of in any other way.

_____ 10. The major obstacle to increasing the percentage of municipal refuse recycled has been the **unwillingness of most people to collect such materials and bring them to collection centers.**

_____ 11. Approximately **30%** of all municipal refuse could easily be composted.

_____ 12. Since implementation of RCRA Subtitle D regulations, there is **little difference in design** between an MSW landfill and a landfill licensed to accept hazardous wastes.

_____ 13. Only wastes categorized as **toxic, corrosive, ignitable, or reactive** are regulated as RCRA hazardous.

_____ 14. Generators of hospital infectious wastes and radioactive wastes **do not have to comply with the RCRA regulations for hazardous waste management.**

_____ 15. The largest portion of hazardous waste managed each year in the U.S. is disposed of by **controlled incineration**.

_____ 16. A person whose health has been damaged by exposure to toxins from a hazardous waste dumpsite **can receive Superfund dollars as compensation**.

_____ 17. States are required to contribute **10%** of the cost of Superfund cleanup projects within their jurisdictions.

_____ 18. It is legal for **householders** to throw out old pesticides, solvents, or other hazardous chemical wastes with their trash.

_____ 19. The intent of recent federal hazardous waste laws is to reduce dependence on landfilling by **strengthening requirements for landfill design (thus making the practice more expensive) and by prohibiting the landfilling of many types of wastes**.

_____ 20. Thanks to the high priority the federal government has given the Superfund program, **progress in cleaning up abandoned waste sites has been rapid** and it is expected that within the next decade the problem will largely have been solved.

C. Fill-in-the-Blank:

_____   1. Approximately how much refuse does the average American throw away each year?

_____   2. Currently, what is the most common method of municipal refuse disposal in the U.S.?

_____   3. Nationally, what percentage of municipal wastes are being recycled/ composted at present?

_____   4. In what way does a bioreactor differ from a conventional sanitary landfill?

_____   5. What type of source separation strategy is being provided by many municipal governments in an effort to make recycling as convenient as possible?

a) _____   6. Name two ways in which sanitary landfilling differs from open dumping.

b) _____

a) _____   7. Cite two approaches to creating greater market demand for recycled materials that state or federal governments are adopting.

b) _____

a) _____   8. List two items that proponents of waste-to-energy incineration cite as advantages over landfilling.

b) _____

a) _____   9. At present, what are the two main environmental concerns with waste-to-energy incineration?

b) _____

_____   10. Give an example of "grasscycling."

a) _____   11. Name two horticultural advantages of using vermicompost as compared with conventional compost.

b) _____

_____   12. Name an element of the municipal waste stream that would be a good target for any serious waste reduction effort.

_____   13. "Reuse and donation" is regarded as the most desirable management option for what component of the municipal waste stream?

a) _____   14. Name two plant species currently being used to remediate contaminated soils.

b) _____

_____   15. What widespread source of hazardous waste problems, found in virtually every community in the U.S., was targeted by regulations promulgated under Subtitle I of RCRA?

_____   16. What type of waste material constitutes the largest portion of the infamous "Great Pacific Garbage Patch"?

_____   17. What is the fastest-growing segment of the North American recycling industry?

_____   18. What major federal environmental law, passed in 1976 and subsequently amended, marked a giant step forward in U.S. efforts to manage currently generated hazardous wastes safely?

_____   19. What problem was the Superfund (CERCLA) intended to solve?

_____   20. Which federal agency has the primary responsibility for promulgating rules and regulations to implement the nation's hazardous waste programs?

D. List the characteristics that the government uses to determine a waste as RCRA hazardous and give an example of a waste that would be included in that category:

                 Waste Characteristic   **Example**

1.

2.

3.

4.

E. Essay:

Explain what is meant by "Pollution Prevention." Why is this concept rapidly gaining acceptance as the best approach to resource management? List some P2 strategies that businesses or industries could adopt to minimize their waste stream.

F. Activity:

Make a survey of your residence, listing all the items which, if discarded, would qualify as "hazardous wastes." How do you generally dispose of these items? Call your City Hall (or mayor, alderman, council member, etc.) and inquire whether a community-wide household hazardous waste collection day has ever been tried or is under consideration. How much support for such an effort do you feel exists in your community?